Essential Oils
for
Beginners

The Complete Guide: Aromatherapy, Essential Oils, and Essential Oils Recipes

Table of Contents

Book Description

Are you sick of seeing advertisements for synthetic, chemical filled products claiming to work miracles?

Well, you can say goodbye to all that.

In this book, I will enlighten you on the true miracle–a natural method that has been used for thousands of years to achieve a multitude of benefits: aromatherapy.

What this book will teach you:

- The basics of essential oils, including its history, production, benefits, method of use, storage, and lots more;
- An informative guide on the most popular essential oils in the market;
- All about carrier oils, their benefits and why they differ from essential oils;
- How to blend essential oils safely, including special tips and precautions;
- Countless recipes for cleaning, illnesses, anti–aging, weight loss, mental wellbeing, pets, cosmetic benefits, insect repellents and so much more!

Read on to change your life for good with essential oils–a true miracle.

Introduction

If you are someone that is looking for a miracle product that will aid you in the majority of household or physical issues that you may be having, then you don't need to look any further.

This guidebook will provide you with a plethora of tips, tricks, recipes and knowledge regarding essential oils—the secret to good health, a better home, and a happier life!

That's right. There are countless numbers of different essential oils out there, each of which has their own extraordinary benefits. They have been used by millions of people for years upon years, and the advantages of using them have been proven by science.

However, it is difficult to know how to use them and how to get started if you are a beginner, and that's why this book is an absolute must—read.

In this book, I will enlighten you about the history of essential oils, as well as what they are, how they are produced and how to get started using them.

After that, we'll discuss all of the most popular and beneficial essential oils available these days, one by one. We'll get into the nitty gritty of carrier oils, how to blend oils, and we'll discuss some amazing recipes that can be used for different issues you may be having with your body or your mind, as well as ones that you can use to create a clean, comfortable and fresh home environment.

You might be a little bit skeptical, and you might doubt the ability of something as natural and simple as essential oils to perform so many amazing things, but it really is true–that's the best part!

To rid yourself of any doubt that you may currently have, just read on and try out all the tips and recipes for yourself, and be prepared to be astounded by the results you'll see.

So, without further ado, let's begin with the very first chapter of the book, in which we'll cover all the basic information you need to be aware of.

Chapter 1 - Essential Oils Basics

In this chapter, we'll discuss the things that are musts for you to know before you get into the blending of essential oils or using them in recipes.

Before you can do that, you need to be very well informed about what essential oils are, how they work, how to use and store them, etc. etc.

The reason for this is because, if you do not educate yourself about these things, there is a possibility that your concoctions of essential oils will be rendered ineffective.

When used in the incorrect manner, essential oils could end up doing more harm than good, which is why I created this chapter to help you prevent that from happening.

You definitely don't want to miss out on all of the miracles that well stored and formulated essential oils can perform!

With that, let's get into the history of essential oils.

History of essential oils

Essential oils were, once upon a time, called 'aromatic oils', and they have been used in many different countries, continents and cultures. Some cultures used them for treating illnesses–something that is still practiced to this day–while others used them for religious ceremonies and other religious purposes.

While the exact year or even the exact century in which the fame of the healing properties of essential oils arose is not known, we do know that, at some point, it did happen. After this, the knowledge of the many benefits of essential oils began to spread to even more countries, even more cultures, making it a global revolution of sorts.

The earliest evidence of the use and knowledge of herbs and plant extracts is provided by cave paintings in a certain region of France, which have been discovered, by carbon dating, to be thousands of years old. These cave paintings suggested that medicinal herbs and the like were used back then.

However, for all we know, they might have been used much before that, too.

So essential oils are by no means a sketchy, newly formulated trick that I am trying to push you. It is something that has been used successfully by many of our ancestors.

In Egypt, essential oils were initially used in ointments, cosmetics, perfumes, medicines and more as early as 4500 B.C.E. When Egypt was at its most powerful, only the high–rank people such as priests and pharaohs were considered worthy of possessing essential oils.

In China, essential oils were first used in around 2600 B.C.E. Huang Ti, the famous emperor of that time, wrote a book on medicine that contained knowledge about essential oils that is still used today!

In Rome, it was quite common for people to apply generous amounts of aromatic oils to their skin, their clothing, as well as to use them for massaging and bathing.

In India, when there was an outbreak of the Bubonic Plague, antibiotics were often replaced by the use of essential oils–a method that was surprisingly successful. In addition to this, essential oils were used for many spiritual and philosophical purposes.

And that is just a tiny fraction of the different areas in which essential oils were used many years ago! Now that you know a little bit about the background of essential oils let's talk about what they are.

What are essential oils?

If you decided to begin this book with no pre–existing knowledge about essential oils, or even an idea as to what they are, then fear not.

I will provide you with some information that will clear up any haziness that you had on the subject.

First, let's talk about the name.

Where did the term 'essential oil' originate from?

Well, it is actually a shortened form of the original name, 'quintessential oil'. This came from the idea of the fifth element of matter, 'quintessence', which was considered to be life force.

Essential oils are basically plant extracts that are removed by physical processes rather than chemical processes.

While they are still within the plants, essential oils help the plant to adapt to its altering environment, as well as a few other purposes such as to attract insects for pollination, to defend against predators (i.e. harmful insects and small animals) as well as to act as an antimicrobial agent.

Essential oils in the plant are released internally via secretory cavities or ducts. Cavities are sphere–shaped spaces while ducts are more extended spaces. Some species of plants posses cavities while others posses ducts.

When it comes to external secretions, plants often have trichomes (hair–like structures on the surface of the plant) to perform this function. Plants with trichomes include the peppermint plant, spearmint plant, and a lavender plant.

That's enough information to give you a clear basic idea about what essential oils are, and the plants that they originate from. Let's move on to the next segment.

How are essential oils produced?

When thinking about how essential oils are removed from plants, you might be imagining a lot of chemical processes used to extract the oils.

While it's true that chemical processes are used by some, the truest forms of essential oils are always extracted by physical methods alone.

The main method is, of course, distillation, which has been used since ancient times. According to research, the extraction of essential oils via steam distillation has been performed for approximately 5000 years.

Even in this modern day and age, distillation is still one of the most efficient and most common ways of extracting essential oils.

During distillation, the plant matter is placed on a grid in a still. The still is closed up, and then steam or water goes through the plant so that its constituents (including the oils) rise into a pipe and then into the condenser. In the condenser, the vapor turns into liquid, which is then collected. The essential oil usually floats on top of the water, making it easy to remove.

Another method that is sometimes used to remove oils from plants is called cold–pressing. Previously, this was a process that was performed by hand via sponge–pressing. These days, however, it is a process that is usually performed by a machine that pricks the plant material (usually the rind of a fruit) to release the essential oil.

Oils that are produced by distillation are not quite as stable as those produced by cold pressing.

When it comes to citrus oils, therefore, it is best to use cold pressed ones for aromatherapy.

Those are the two main methods of producing essential oils. Both processes have their disadvantages and advantages, but it is generally fine to use oils from either one of the processes.

In the next segment, we'll get into how essential oils work.

How do essential oils work?

In this segment, I will talk about how essential oils work when it comes to your body.

So, you see, there are a number of ways by which essential oils may be taken into your body.

The first way is by application to the skin. The second way is by inhalation, and the third by ingestion.

When it comes to your skin, many people seem unsure of how, exactly, essential oils can cure problems with bones or muscles via application to the skin.

Well, you need to be aware of the fact that your skin is permeable, to some extent. So the chemicals in the essential oils can be absorbed by the skin in the same way that the medicinal creams you buy from the drugstore are absorbed.

Certain factors can increase the absorption, e.g. heat or application to certain parts of the body (such as soles of the feet or palms of the hand).

Now, let's talk about inhalation, which can be done with the mouth or the nose. Inhaling certain essential oils can, in fact, cure some particular bodily issues.

An example of this is that peppermint oil can reduce the nauseous feeling that you may get from car sickness, sea sickness, pregnancy, etc.

The reason for this is that when you inhale, the molecules of the essential oil that enter your nose react with your brain, triggering certain feelings or emotions. This is why essential oils are also commonly used to treat stress and anxiety, as well as depression.

When it comes to ingestion, you have to be very careful. There are certain essential oils that can cause toxic reactions in the liver, which is why ingestion is not the best method to reap the benefits of essential oils unless it is something that has been prescribed by a professional.

Now, let's move on to talk about what aromatherapy is and what it involves.

What is aromatherapy?

Seeing as how aromatherapy uses essential oils, it is also often called 'essential oil therapy'. This is more than just a simple process like brushing your teeth or combing your hair–it is an art, and it takes knowledge and practice to perform correctly. This book is what will provide you with the knowledge you need, but practice is something you will need to do on your own.

It is an art that is meant to boost not only the health of your body but the health of your mind and your spirit so that you can live your life with all these aspects working correctly and in harmony with each other.

The name 'aromatherapie' was created in the 1930s by the French chemist called Gattefosse. He even wrote a book called 'Gatefosse's Aromatherapy' in which he wrote about how essential oils could be used to cure a number of different bodily issues.

By the term 'aromatherapy' you would think that any good smelling item such as a flower or an aerosol air freshener could work, but that simply is not the case. In fact, many essential oils with great benefits do not even smell pleasant, which makes the term 'aromatherapy' quite a confusing one!

True aromatherapy is when you make use of essential oils by application, inhalation or (less commonly) ingestion in a therapeutic and relaxing manner.

So, now that you have an idea about what aromatherapy is let's talk about the benefits of aromatherapy and essential oils in general.

Benefits and uses of aromatherapy and essential oils

There are a vast number of superb benefits and uses of essential oils, and the fact that aromatherapy is such a widely used technique is proof of this fact–after all, why would something ineffective be touted by so many people, all over the world?

That's just it–it wouldn't be. So, in this segment, we'll go over only a small portion of the countless uses and benefits that aromatherapy and essential oils can have.

Essential oils such as those derived from black pepper can be used as muscle relaxants for those that suffer from soreness. Oils extracted from lavender are one of the few kinds of oils that do not require dilution, and can be used to help repair injured cells of the body, while oils from grapefruit can help to detox the body of harmful waste materials.

Chamomile essential oil is an anti–inflammatory, anti–allergenic oil that can be used to treat skin issue and also has a relaxing effect when inhaled.

Peppermint oil, apart from being able to help with nausea, can be used to help with a congested nose or to aid in digestive issues. It can even be applied to the temples and massaged there to relieve severe headaches.

Bergamot oil, believe it or not, can actually help fight depression and can also help with inflammation, both external and internal.

Tea tree oil is anti bacterial and anti fungal and is commonly used to successfully treat the irksome skin condition that is acne.

Rosemary oil is a pain relieving oil that can also help to stimulate the circulation of blood.

Eucalyptus oil is yet another antibacterial and antiviral oil and is also one that can be used as a decongestant. If you are having issues with a cough and a stuffy nose, eucalyptus oil is the one to go for.

Those are a few of the countless uses of essential oils–if I tried to elaborate on the uses of every single type of oil out there, I'd be going on for ages!

For those that want to know more, don't worry. We will have an entire chapter later on in the book to summarize the uses of the most common essential oils.

How to use essential oils

In this particular segment, we'll talk about the methods by which you can use essential oils. As you should know by now, essential oils can be inhaled, topically applied or ingested, in some cases.

However, you need to know more than that if you wish to use aromatherapy in your daily life. You need to know how to apply the oils topically, how to inhale them. We won't get into the details about ingestion because, as I said earlier, it is a process that is not to be done unless recommended by your doctor.

In order to choose the best method for you, you need to check if the essential oil in question is one that is irritating when topically applied to the skin. If so, you have two options. You can either dilute it down to a concentration that is not irritating at all, or you can go for the inhalation technique instead.

Also, you should know that aromatherapy for healing wounds and external injuries is nearly always achieved by topical application. Boosting your emotions or mood can be done by the topical application, but inhalation is a quicker method to achieve results.

Baths with essential oils will have an effect by both inhalation and absorption through the skin.

Now, let's talk about the methods of inhalation.

One option is to use a diffuser. This is a device in which essential oils are placed, often diluted with water. Sometimes heat is used, depending on your particular diffuser, and the essential oil will evaporate and diffuse throughout the air. Some diffusers run for a certain period of time and then automatically turn off while others require manual switching off.

Dry evaporation is another method that can be used. In this method, a few drops of the oil are put on a tissue paper. For gentle exposure, all you do is wait for the evaporation to occur so that you can inhale small amounts of the oil.

For a more intense exposure, you may bring the tissue right in front of your nose–however, be aware that certain essential oils can be very strong.

Steam can also be used to aid you in inhaling essential oils. All you need to do is put a few drops of the oil into a bowl of hot, steaming water, which will rapidly cause the oil to turn into vapor. You can even cover your head and face, as well as the bowl, with a cloth or towel and then inhale from under the towel. In this case, you will also have to take care that the mixture is not too strong.

The last method that can be used is a spray. You need to mix a few drops of your chosen oil with a solution that is water soluble, shake it and then spray it in the air. This is an easy way to inhale essential oils and perk up your mood.

Now let's talk about topical application.

When you apply essential oils topically, you need to use carrier oils–something we'll discuss in detail in a later chapter. For now, let's just go over the techniques.

One method that is semi–topical is gargling. You mix a few drops of the oil in water and then gargle for a few minutes, taking special care not to swallow the solution. This can be a method of topical application for issues that you might have with your throat, e.g. a sore throat.

Another method is, of course, bathing. A few drops of essential oils can be mixed into your bath before you get in, and bath salts can be used to help the essential oil disperse. By doing this, you will have the benefits of the topical application as well as inhalation!

A compress is also a good way to use essential oils topically. All you do is dilute the oil with a carrier (read chapter 3 for more on carriers) and then apply it to a dressing, which can be then applied on the required area. You may accompany this with heat. This is great for sore muscles, stiff joints, etc.

The last method of topical application is one of the most popular: a massage. Massages are adored by millions of people and using essential oils in conjunction with a massage is extremely beneficial. You just need to mix a few drops of the essential oil with a carrier and then rub into the skin, or have someone else rub it into the skin.

And that's all there is to know about the basics of how to use essential oils. Next, we'll talk about how to buy and store them.

How to buy and store essential oils

In this segment, I'll inform you about the little tips you need to be aware of to help you purchase the best quality essential oils possible. If you buy poor quality essential oils, you will not see any of the benefits that we've discussed earlier, which is why this knowledge is so important.

Essential oils with other substances mixed in them can, in fact, do harm to your body.

First of all, if you are looking at an oil that claims to be a fragrance or perfume oil, put it down immediately. These terms should be a dead giveaway that the oil is not a pure one and has added chemicals in it.

Secondly, if the oil is packaged in a plastic or glass container that is see–through, proceed with caution. Most legitimate aromatherapy oils are packaged in small, dark colored bottles.

Another tip to be aware of is that if you are shopping online, don't be afraid to contact the company and present them with any questions you have regarding the details of the oils they are selling.

When buying in stores, make sure that the bottles are properly sealed and do not look old (e.g. dented boxes, dusty bottles) as this can mean that the essential oil is not fit for use.

You should also be aware that organic oils are far better for you than non–organic oils. That's not to say that nonorganic oils are bad, but they do not have quite as many benefits as organic oils do.

If you are trying out a particular brand of essential oils for the first time, don't go overboard. Start with a small, sample sized product and only buy more if you believe that the product was exceptionally good.

Those are all the most important things to be aware of when it comes to purchasing essential oils. Next, let's talk about the things you need to know about storing essential oils.

Proper storage of essential oils is of the utmost importance, and it can play a huge part in how long they last.

As you now know, essential oils should always be in dark containers–this is so that they block out UV rays because UV rays can shorten the shelf life of essential oils.

In addition to this, make sure you store the bottles in a dark area where the sunlight does not shine. This will prevent oxidation.

Citrus oils, in particular, oxidize very easily, so it is best to keep them in the refrigerator at a temperature between 6–10 degrees Celsius. Excessive heat is not a good idea for any type of essential oil. In the summers, it is fine to store essential oils other than citrus ones in the fridge, as well.

Another thing to be careful about when storing essential oils is that they remain out of the reach of any children or pets you might have. Large quantities of the essential oil could be harmful, not to mention the glass of the bottles that could be broken.

Lastly, be sure to never, ever transfer your essential oils (unless they are highly diluted) into plastic containers, as the oils can actually break down the plastic.

That's all for this segment. Let's move on to the safety and precautionary tips in the next segment.

Safety tips and precautions

Essential oils may seem like a harmless thing that you would not have to be careful around, but that is not the case at all.

In fact, essential oils can be dangerous, sometimes even fatal if they are misused. That's why I am dedicating a segment to enlightening you about the precautions you need to take regarding essential oils.

First, as I said earlier, keep them away from children and pets. That's an absolute must. Secondly, if used on infants, essential oils must only be used in extremely dilute solutions so as not to harm the sensitive skin of the infant.

Some oils, especially citrus oils, are phototoxic. This means that you will need to avoid sun exposure on the day you apply these to your skin in order to avoid sun damage or sun burns.

If you have any allergies, then be extra careful when using essential oils. Test them out on a small area of the skin and make sure no irritation occurs before using them all over the body.

You absolutely need to keep away any kind of essential oils from flames, as many of them are highly flammable and could cause fatal accidents.

Essential oils that have not been diluted should never come anywhere near sensitive areas of the body or the mucous membranes.

If you have been using a number of synthetic products on certain areas of your face or body, take special care when applying essential oils to that area.

Those are the major precautions to know before attempting to use essential oils on yourself or anyone else.

In the next chapter, we will go over all of the major, popular essential oils in alphabetical order, as well as a few of each of their uses.

Chapter 2 - The Most Popular Essential Oils

If an interest about essential oils has been sparked within you, but you aren't quite sure which oils to buy and which ones are suitable for your situation or your problems, then this is the chapter for you.

We'll go over each commonly used essential oil one by one and describe what it can do for you.

Without further ado, let's get into it.

Bergamot

This particular essential oil is a citrus scented one that comes from the Citrus Beragamia tree, which is common in Southeast Asia but can now be found in many other parts of the world. This oil is commonly used in perfumes, as well as in aromatherapy.

The cold pressing technique is performed on the rind of the bergamot fruit in order to extract the oil. This oil can be used via inhalation with a diffuser, or it can be used in one's bath or as a massage oil (when mixed with a few other oils).

Bergamot oil can help with stress, lack of appetite, depression, as well as certain infections of the skin.

It can also stimulate the digestive system and improve the mood of those that are sickly.

It is necessary to apply this to the skin only in a very diluted form so as not to irritate or burn the skin. Sunlight must be avoided directly after application.

Carrot seed

Carrot seed oil is extracted by steam distillation of, of course, carrot seeds.

The best quality of this essential oil is its astounding antioxidant content. Because of these antioxidants, carrot seed oil can help you look and feel younger by protecting your skin from wrinkling, preventing your hair from prematurely turning white, and preventing your eyesight from deteriorating.

In addition to this, this oil can prevent certain types of cancer.

Carrot seed oil is also a detoxifier which can help clean out your system, and it is also a diuretic.

This essential oil is safe to use during pregnancy, with caution.

Cedarwood

Cedarwood oil is an essential oil with a musky scent that comes from the Juniperus Virginiana tree-one that is common in North America. This oil is one that has been used for many, many years. It was even used in ancient Egypt and is, quite possibly, one of the first essential oils ever used.

This oil is produced by distillation from woodchips of the tree. The oil has a distinctive yellow color, and can be used by inhalation or as a constituent of massage oil, or even applied on the face by mixing it with a facial cream.

This particular oil has a calming quality to it and can help with stress and mood swings. It is beneficial for the skin, too.

This oil, however, is best avoided during pregnancy, and should never be used in highly concentrated solutions.

Chamomile

Chamomile oil is one of the most popular essential oils there is. It is well known for being used in tea, as well as for its calming and soothing characteristics. The leaves of the chamomile plant are used to extract the oil via distillation.

There are two varieties of chamomile (Roman and German), and the oils of each variety have very similar benefits.

Chamomile can be used in massage oils, in a diffuser for inhalation or for steam therapy. It is also commonly used by mixing with lotions to be applied topically.

Chamomile is, as I said, great for calming and relaxing. It is a proven mood enhancer and anti-depressant. It is also antibacterial, which is a plus for infections.

Both varieties of chamomile are great for inflammation and skin issues such as acne.

This is another oil that is not to be used during pregnancy.

Cinnamon

Cinnamon is a spice that all of us have heard of and/ or consumed at some point or the other. Cinnamon oil, however, is something different. It is obtained from the bark and leaves of the cinnamon tree via distillation.

It has been used as a tonic and a digestive aid for many years, and it has a very distinct, sharp smell.

It has a number of benefits, such as promoting circulation within the body as well as on the skin, promoting the immune system, boosting oral health, alleviating soreness, etc.

In addition to all of these physical benefits, it is a known mood enhancer, which is a big plus for those dealing with depression and anxiety.

It is also great to consume in tiny amounts, and has a distinct, pleasant spicy flavor.

Apart from this, it is great to inhale or even apply topically once diluted.

It must be used with caution by pregnant women.

Clary sage

Clary sage oil is extracted via steam distillation of the clary sage plant's buds and leaves.

The health benefits of this oil include the fact that it is a potent antidepressant, as well as a sedative.

It has astringent properties which can greatly benefit the skin, and it may also be used to create a natural deodorant.

One of the best uses of this oil is that it can treat wounds due to its antibacterial and antiseptic nature.

Pregnant women must use this with caution.

Clove

Clove oil is one that has been used for over 2000 years, and is one of the most well known and most commonly used oils out there.

It is the dried bud of the clove flower that is distilled in order to create clove oil.

Clove oil is best known for its benefits for the teeth and mouth-it can alleviate toothaches, soothe the gums and can counteract throat pain. This makes it great for respiratory issues, too.

It is best applied topically after being diluted properly, and it may even be ingested in tiny amounts-e.g. a drop in a cup of herbal tea-to help with nausea. For respiratory issues, steaming or using a diffuser may help.

Due to its numbing nature, it is also known to be able to relieve aches and muscle pains.

Due to its potency, however, it absolutely needs to be diluted before any kind of use, and is best avoided by pregnant women.

Cypress

Cypress oil is obtained through steam distillation of young twigs, stems and needles of the Cypress tree.

One of the most important benefits of this oil is that it is a diuretic. This is significant because it helps to eliminate all the toxins and excess fat that may do harm to your body.

By doing this, cypress oil not only detoxes your body, it also helps you to lose excess weight.

In addition to this, cypress oil is antispasmodic and may also be used as a respiratory tonic to increase the efficiency of the lungs.

It is best avoided by pregnant women.

Eucalyptus

Eucalyptus oil is an oil that is extracted from leaves or twigs of the Eucalyptus tree, which is commonly found in Australia, by distillation. This particular oil has a distinctive, strong scent, and is considered to be good for enhancing one's concentrating power and curing or relieving respiratory issues. It is also used as an antiseptic, and can be great for relieving a stuffy nose.

Due to the cooling sensation it provides on the skin, it can help relieve the symptoms of fevers and can fight the pain of headaches, as well as relieve sore muscles and achy joints, to some extent. In addition to that, its scent is great for getting rid of unpleasant odors.

Ingesting this oil in large, concentrated amounts, however, is extremely dangerous-it can even cause death.

Pregnant women should avoid this oil, and cautions should be taken if one is breastfeeding.

Ginger

Ginger is a very common product used in cooking, especially in Asian culture, and has many health benefits. Its oil, however, is something that has innumerable benefits.

Ginger oil is extracted from the ginger plant by distillation, and is a great digestive aid. It also has antiseptic and anti-inflammatory properties, making it great for skincare.

It is even known to boost the health of your heart and relieve stress!

This oil can be applied topically after dilution, and is great to inhale in a bath, by a diffuser, etc. to relieve stress, too.

It is another oil that is good for ingestion in tiny amounts when it comes to treating stomach problems. Too much of it is not a good idea, though!

Grapefruit

Grapefruit is a delicious sweet and tart fruit that many of us enjoy eating on hot summer days.

Grapefruit oil is extracted by cold pressing the peel, and it has a sharp and refreshing smell, just as most citrus oils do.

The properties of grapefruit oil include the fact that it is a diuretic, a disinfectant, an antiseptic, antidepressant and a tonic.

This means it is great for acne prone skin via topical application, massages or bathing, and can be used to inhale or ingest in small amounts.

The only precaution to take is to stay out of sunlight after external use-this is the same for all citrus oils, as well.

Care must be taken by pregnant women.

Helichrysum

Helichrysum oil is extracted from the helichrysum flower, and it is a costly and rare oil with a remarkably long shelf life.

The benefits of this oil can be attributed to its antiallergenic, anticoagulant and anti-inflammatory properties.

Because this oil is an anticoagulant, it can help to save lives. This oil can be a great help for people who are at a high risk of heart attacks due to having a high cholesterol content in their blood, as it helps to thin the blood.

The fact that this oil is antiallergenic is also a huge plus, as it can minimize the unpleasant symptoms of an allergic reaction.

This oil is best avoided by pregnant women.

Jasmine

Jasmine oil comes from the pleasantly scented evergreen 'Jasminum grand forum' which is very common in China. This oil is a bit pricier than a lot of other oils, and this may be because of its rather complicated and unusual extraction method.

Jasmine oil is extracted by a method called solvent extraction, which is rarely performed for other oils.

The process takes several days to be completed and produces much less oil for the amount of work you put into the extraction.

This oil is great to add to bathwater or mix into a concoction of massage oils.

Jasmine oil is said to be a wonderful way to aid individuals suffering from depression, as well as to reduce stress and anxiety. It can also be used to relieve respiratory issues.

This oil is one of the more safe ones to use, but should still be used with caution, especially if pregnant.

Juniper

Juniper oil is extracted through steam distillation of the needles, wood and powdered fruits of juniper.

It used in many industries all over the world, and is also used to flavor certain alcoholic drinks.

The health benefits of the oil include the fact that it is antirheumatic. This is because it helps improve blood circulation and remove toxins, which help fight rheumatism, arthritis, gout and other ailments which are caused by improper circulation.

Juniper oil is also effective on nearly all types of cramps, as well as spasmodic cholera and any spasm causing problems.

Because it is an astringent, Juniper oil can also benefit the skin and teeth and gums.

The oil must be used carefully by pregnant women.

Lavender

Lavender oil is very popular oil in the market these days. The smell alone is a good enough reason to buy it, really!

However, it has a lot more going for it than just its pleasant smell-it is a known stress reliever and is great for those with minor infections such as the flu.

This oil is extracted by distillation of the Lavender flowers. It is best used in bathwater, or for a relaxing massage. It can be inhaled with the help of a diffuser.

Using this on your pillows and bed sheets can also be a great way to prevent or rid yourself of insomnia.

Lavender oil is also an effective antiseptic and is known to be an anti-depressant. In addition to that, it is also one of those oils that can deodorize nasty scents and help with external inflammation of the skin.

Just be sure to watch out if you notice an allergic reaction, and then stop using it.

Lemon

Lemon is, of course, a favorite of many people when it comes to essential oils. This may be because of its tangy and appealing scent.

Lemon oil is known to help sharpen the mind and your concentrating power, as well as to treat skin infections (including acne). It can also help with better digestion as well as with achy joints.

Lemon oil is extracted from the fruit's rind by cold pressing, a method that I described in an earlier chapter.

This oil is great to use as an air freshener due to its fresh and clean smell. This can be done by using a diffuser or a spray.

It can also be mixed into a number of other oils for a great smelling massage oil. Adding it to bath water is also an effective method for this oil.

Lemon oil boosts circulation helps with skin irritation and can smooth your skin. It can also give your immune system a great boost, believe it or not.

Mild to moderate headaches and fevers can be alleviated with lemon oil, and it can also be used to improve your mood.

A few things to keep in mind include the fact that lemon can cause sunburn if you step into sunlight after using it on the skin. In addition to that, it can cause an allergic reaction in certain people, so be sure to perform a patch test.

Lemongrass oil

Lemon oil and lemongrass oil are not the same thing, contrary to what a lot of people seem to think.

To extract this oil, steam distillation of the lemongrass is performed.

This oil is one that is fit be consumed-in small amounts, of course-in food, tea, etc. as well as inhaled or used on the skin.

It is anti microbial and antiseptic, which is a plus for those with acne, and it has anti-depressant properties, too. It is also known to be a deodorizing and sedative product.

Lastly, it is also great for muscle and joint pains, as well as toothaches.

Mandarin

Mandarin oil is extracted from the fruit rind by cold compression.

Apart from being used as a flavoring agent in the food and beverage industry, it has various medicinal benefits as well.

For one thing, it is antiseptic. This means that it can be used to treat wounds, injuries and any bacterial issues.

It is also antispasmodic. A spasm in the respiratory system can cause breathing difficulties, whereas a spasm in the muscles can cause painful cramps. To prevent or eliminate these issues, this oil is a good option to consider.

Mandarin oil is also used to boost the circulation of blood and lymph, especially below the skin to keep it looking young and fresh.

This oil also has the ability to cure digestive problems if it is consumed in small quantities after each meal. It does this by stimulating the production of digestive issues.

Mandarin oil is safe to be consumed by pregnant women in small quantities.

Marjoram

Marjoram oil is touted by many for its ability to calm down people with too much energy, as well as to relieve excessive stress and anxiety.

It can also help with digestive issues, stomach aches, and was often used in medicines in the ancient times.

This oil is produced by extraction from the leaves of the herb, and then distillation.

This oil is great for inhalation by using a diffuser, as it can help with stuffy noses, asthma, and other respiratory ailments.

It can also be added to bathwater to help you get a good night's sleep, and can be mixed with other oils to function as a massage oil-this will help with circulation of blood, and will help you get rid of stress, headaches and lots of other issues.

Marjoram is great for any issues you may be having with circulation, and is also a big help for people suffering from depression.

Keep in mind, however, that this oil is not ideal for pregnant women.

Myrrh oil

Myrrh oil is extracted from the resin. This oil is touted for its many health benefits which can be attributed to its antimicrobial, astringent, antiseptic and immunity boosting properties.

Myrrh essential oil is also great to fight against coughs and colds due to the fact that it has the ability to kill the viruses that cause these issues.

In addition to this, it is also useful for boosting the overall health of your stomach.

Nutmeg

Nutmeg oil is extracted from the seed of the nutmeg tree fruit, which is a huge tree that can grow to be upto 70 feet tall.

Nutmeg oil is very useful in treating muscular pain and join pain. This is due to the fact that it is a sedative.

Nutmeg oil also has anti-inflammatory properties, so it can be massaged into any inflamed area can benefit people with arthritis, rheumatism, etc.

Cramps and indigestion are common issues that can easily be cured by inhaling this oil, or consuming it in small amounts.

In addition to this, nutmeg oil can boost blood circulation amd aid respiratory issues.

Orange oil (sweet)

This is another oil that is produced by cold pressing the rind of the delicious fruit.

Like most citrus oils, it is great for the skin—especially dull or acne prone skin—as well as digestion and infections such as the flu.

This oil can be diluted and applied to the neck and chest area for infections, as well as to the face. It can be inhaled via steaming or diffusing, and can be massaged or added to bath water as well.

Ingestion should be performed with caution, and in tiny amounts.

Some people are prone to irritation from citrus oils, so be sure to perform a patch test before using properly.

Oregano oil

The essential oil of oregano is extracted through steam distillation of fresh oregano leaves.

Along with having antimicrobial and antifungal properties, this oil has medicinal uses as well.

It is an anti-inflammatory, and it can help treat a number of respiratory issues, as well as digestive issues.

One of the most celebrated benefits of oregano oil is the fact that it has some remarkable antioxidants which can benefit the body in numerous ways.

This oil is best when inhaled or applied topically.

Some people are prone to irritation from citrus oils, so be sure to perform a patch test before using properly.

Patchouli

This oil is another one that is very well known. It is popular for its mood enhancing characteristics and its use in skincare.

It comes from the leaves of the Pogostemon cablin plant, and the extract is distillated.

This oil can be added to bathwater or can be inhaled by using a diffuser. It is great for sufferers of anxiety or depression, and can be used topically by mixing with lotions or the like to help with infections of the skin and to heal any external injuries.

It is a very thick oil and is great for increasing the growth of skin cells, smoothing down uneven skin texture, reduce bloating and can even reduce the appearance of cellulite with regular use!

This oil is a strong one, so should be used in small amounts, and with great caution.

Peppermint

Ah, peppermint. One of the most popular essential oils of all, and for good reason.

The cooling and pleasant tingling feeling that peppermint oil can provide is known to help with a concentration of the mind and boosting energy.

Peppermint extract is taken from the herb and then distillated. It is used in lots of skincare creams and lotions for the body and is even used in things like toothpaste.

Peppermint oil can also help reduce irritation of the skin and can reduce a stuffy nose and aid digestive issues.

It should be noted that some people tolerate peppermint poorly when it is applied to the skin, and it can also cause severe stinging if it enters the eyes.

Small children should not be allowed near this oil, and it is best avoided by pregnant women.

Pine

Pine oil is obtained from, of course, the pine tree.

The health benefits of this oil are due to its antibacterial, analgesic and energizing properties.

For one thing, this is a great oil to use for skincare, especially if your skin is prone to rashes or acne. This oil can balance your skin out, leaving it smooth and renewed.

The antioxidant content of this oil also helps to keep your skin young and fresh.

Pine oil can also boost your metabolism and help treat intestinal problems, which can be beneficial for people wishing to lose weight or just improve their overall health.

This oil is also useful for relieving joint pain due to its analgesic nature.

As for emotional benefits, pine oil can create an energized feeling within people and remove stress.

Rose

Rose oil is an absolute must have for a lot of women, mainly because of its feminine and appealing scent. Rose oil is an oil that has been used for many years, and it is more expensive than a lot of oils, not because of the method being difficult but because of a lot of roses that are required to produce the oil.

Rose oil is removed from the petals of the flower and is then distilled to get rose oil.

Rose oil can help with depression, anxiety and can aid indigestion. It improves circulation of blood and can even relieve symptoms of respiratory problems.

It is also great for the skin and makes it smell lovely.

This oil is not a particularly dangerous one, but it still bests to be cautious when pregnant.

Rosemary

Rosemary oil is well known for its ability to sharpen concentration and help clear up the mind. This herb is one that was once considered to be almost sacred due to its many benefits.

Rosemary oil is extracted from the herb when it is flowering. This extract is distillated. You can add rosemary oil in your diffuser or humidifier to help with a stuffy nose or other respiratory issues, and you can add it to your massage oils if you have achy joints or sore muscles, as well as any digestive issues.

Rosemary oil can also be added to hair products to stimulate circulation to the scalp and increase the growth of hair.

It has even been thought to improve memory and improve the overall performance of your brain, making it great to use when studying for a test!

It can be massaged into the temples for headaches and can be used to treat a variety of skin issues, too. It is an antiseptic, which means it can help treat quite a few infections.

Individuals with high blood pressure or those that are pregnant should avoid the use of this essential oil.

Sandalwood

Sandalwood oil is another very common essential oil.

It has this distinctive woody fragrance to it which makes it easy to identify, and it is a rather expensive one, too.

The best time to extract this oil from the tree is when the tree is fully mature. This takes quite a bit of time, limiting the amount of oil you can get. This is probably the reason for its high price.

Sandalwood oil, like many others, is produced by extraction followed by distillation. This oil can be used as one of many oils in a massage oil mixture, it can be mixed into skincare lotions and it can be put into a diffuser. In diluted form, it is also good for gargling.

Sandalwood oil can help with infections of the urinary tract, and can also be used to alleviate pain in the chest. It is also one of those oils that has soothing properties, which means it can reduce stress and anxiety.

It also hydrates skin and prevents and reduces inflammation.

Tangerine

Tangerines are extremely healthy fruits, and they provide us with a number of beneficial properties through their oils!

This cold pressed oil (produced from the rind of the fruit) can be used as an antiseptic, a sedative, and antispasmodic and can also be used to boost cell regeneration!

This means it is best applied topically after dilution, or inhales via steaming, diffusing or bathing. Ingestion is not recommended, although it is not harmful in small amounts.

Caution must be taken by pregnant women, and it should not be used before sun exposure.

Tea tree

Tea tree oil is something that I am sure many acne sufferers have heard about, and for good reason-tea tree oil has antibacterial properties, which means it is a great way to treat acne.

It is also known to boost the immune system and reduce infections.

Tea tree oil is extracted from the leaves of the tree and then distillated. It can be inhaled by the steam inhalation method or with a diffuser, but it is best when applied topically to the body.

You can mix it into lotions or creams or your massage oils to rub into the skin. You can even add it to your bath, or to your shampoo to make use of its healing abilities.

Tea tree oil truly has countless benefits. It can be used to repel insects, to help heal external wounds, it can help with an array of skin conditions, it can reduce muscle soreness or joint aches, it can soothe burns and treat respiratory conditions, as well as so much more.

The only precautions to take are to avoid using it too close to the eyes or the nose.

Valerian

Valerian is a perennial flower native to parts of Asia and Europe, and is now grown in several other places.

Valerian oil is well known across the globe for its amazing benefits, such as being able to aid sleep disorders, anxiety, depression, stomach issues, blood pressure and make the skin glow.

It is a great oil to consume in tiny amounts, but keep in mind that excessive consumption can be harmful to the health.

In addition to this, you may want to think about inhaling it for sleep disorders, or diluting and applying to skin.

Vanilla

Vanilla essential oil is obtained by solvent extraction of a substance obtained from vanilla beans that have been fermented. These beans come from the vanilla plant.

Now, when you think of vanilla, you think of ice cream. Pudding. Cookies. All kinds of delicious things.

Vanilla oil is something that is not as unhealthy as any of those items, though!

Vanilla oil has some amazing antioxidant properties, making it able to protect the body from cancer, as well as improving your immune system. It is also a sedative and an antidepressant, making it a good choice for those that want to boost their mood or get a better night's sleep.

In addition to this, it can also help fight infections-and it smells absolutely lovely, too!

You may consume this in small amounts, but it is best applied topically or inhaled via bathwater, diffusing, steaming, etc. I would recommend using it in baths due to its relaxing scent.

Yarrow

Yarrow oil is extracted by steam distillation of the plant, and has a vast number of health benefits, of which I will name a few.

It is a popular antiseptic that is included in quite a few antiseptic creams that you may see in stores-this means it's good for wounds or any sort of skin infection, including acne.

It can also be used as a digestive aid for those that suffer from indigestion, and can be tranquilizing, helping those with insomnia or other sleep issues.

Lastly, it is antispasmodic and anti-inflammatory, too!

Ingestion should be avoided when pregnant.

Ylang-Ylang

Ylang-ylang oil has a distinctive sweet smell which is known to help with stress.

This oil is taken from the flowers of a tropical tree, after which it is distillated. As is the case with so many other oils, Ylang-ylang can be used in a diffuser, in lotions or for massaging and baths.

It can be used to help with headaches, queasiness of the stomach, it can increase hair growth, treat skin problems and regulate blood pressure.

It is fairly safe oil, but large amounts could be overwhelming due to the fragrance.

That concludes this chapter on all of the most popular essential oils that are used these days. By using the information in this chapter, you can decide which essential oils are the best for your particular situation, and you can go ahead and purchase those oils.

In the next chapter, we will talk about carrier oils, something that I have mentioned a couple of times already.

This is something that you absolutely need to know about if you wish to use the technique of aromatherapy, so be sure to read on carefully.

Chapter 3 - Carrier Oils Basics

In this chapter, we'll get into each and every detail that you need to know about carrier oils. Essential oils can't be properly used without them, making them an extremely important part of the aromatherapy process.

We'll begin by discussing what, exactly, they are.

What are carrier oils?

If you have absolutely no idea as to what carrier oils are, let me explain it to you in a simple manner.

You see, if you apply essential oils directly to your skin, they are likely to cause irritation or unpleasant reactions. Carrier oils can be used to dilute essential oils, making them gentler on the skin.

The reason that they are called 'carrier oils' is because of the fact that they help carry the essential oils through the skin.

Most carrier oils are fatty oils such as coconut oil, avocado oil, etc.

Like essential oils, carrier oils also have their own benefits for the skin and body, and can have a number of different therapeutic effects.

The fact that most carrier oils are highly moisturizing is also an added bonus-this is why these fatty oils are often used in moisturizers, skin care products, lip balms, hair products and the like.

We'll get more in-depth with the benefits of carrier oils in another segment of this chapter.

For now, let's move on to discuss the methods by which carrier oils are produced.

How are carrier oils produced?

Just like essential oils, carrier oils are also extracted by a number of different methods, some of which are very similar to the extraction methods of essential oils.

One of these methods is cold pressing, which I described earlier. The fatty segment of the botanical is mechanically pressed to receive the oil. This method must be performed at a temperature at or below 120 degrees, otherwise it is known as being expeller pressed.

Expeller pressed oils are also obtained by mechanically pressing the botanical, although this method requires high pressure if you wish to obtain the maximum amount of product possible

Solvent extraction is also a method that I briefly mentioned in the previous chapter. At times, it is necessary to use some sort of solvent to extract the oil of certain seeds, nuts, etc.

Once the oil is extracted, the solvent is removed. A tiny amount of it may still remain in the oil, though.

CO_2 extraction is also fairly common. In this method, fluid carbon dioxide (created by the use of high pressure) is used as a solvent. This allows the desirable part of the plant to be extracted without having to worry about the degradation that can be caused from heat. Once the procedure is complete, the pressure can be released. The carbon dioxide then immediately returns to gaseous state.

That sums up a few of the major methods of extraction and production of carrier oils.

Carrier oils vs. essential oils

A lot of people find it confusing to differentiate between carrier oils and essential oils, and they don't understand what makes these two types of oils belong to separate categories rather than be grouped into one big category.

Read on and your confusion will be no more.

First of all, carrier oils are usually vegetable oils that are derived from the fatty portion of the plant e.g. the seed, nut or kernel. Essential oils, however, come from areas like the bark, the root, the stem or the leaf or the flowers.

Secondly, carrier oils are not particularly strong and concentrated. They can be applied directly to the skin, and will cause no irritation, stinging or burning. In contrast to this, essential oils are extremely potent. A generous and concentrated application can cause some serious discomfort and harm, even with the milder varieties of oils.

Another difference between the two types of oils is the amount that you need to use. Since carrier oils are quite good for the skin and hair, large amounts of this can be used. Essential oils have their benefits too, but must be used in tiny quantities due to their potency.

Carrier oils do not degrade at all, and they require quite a bit of heat to evaporate. Essential oils degrade in the presence of excessive heat or light, though, and they evaporate instantaneously when left in the open.

Lastly, carrier oils are rather thick and sticky while essential oils are thin and watery.

Those are the major differences between the two types of oils.

General benefits of using carrier oils

Just like essential oils, carrier oils have multitudes of benefits, which is one of the reasons why it is such a great idea to mix the two and get the best of both worlds.

Carrier oils from different seeds and nuts have different benefits, but a lot of them are similar, too.

Some of these benefits include the fact that most carrier oils are highly moisturizing and are great for softening skin and hair.

These moisturizing properties can, in term, help to prevents wrinkles, can reduce the appearance of scars and cellulite, etc.

A benefit that I already mentioned is, of course, the fact that carrier oils are what allow essential oils to penetrate through the skin. If you did not use carrier oils, you would be missing out on all of the amazing benefits of essential oils for your skin, too!

So, yes, carrier oils have a whole lot of benefits that you absolutely need to reap by mixing them with essential oils.

For more specific details about the benefits of particular carrier oils, move on to the next segment.

Popular carrier oils + individual benefits

In this final segment, we'll briefly discuss the benefits of some of the most popular kinds of carrier oils.

This will make it easier for you to pick which ones would be best for you, personally, to use.

Almond oil is one of the most popular oils around-sweet almond oil in particular. It contains vitamins A, B, E as well as protein and calcium and lots of other great nutrients that will benefit the skin. This oil is one that is well known for its ability to reduce the appearance of wrinkles, as well as to help the skin retain moisture.

Apricot kernel oil is an oil which is derived from the kernel of the apricort fruit. This oil contains lots of potassium, protein, vitamins A, C and E. Popular carrier oil with anti-wrinkle and antioxidant properties. When combined with essential oils, this oil can deliver numerous benefits to the skin and body, making it a great pick as a carrier oil.

Argan oil is an extremely popular oil which is used by many people to restore moisture in the skin and hair. The claims made about this oil are all justified, as it contains vitamin E, Carotenes, Squalenes and other nutrients that are extremely hydrating and are great to reduce stretch marks and wrinkles.

Avocado oil is derived from the avocado fruit which is rich in healthy fats and nutrients. With its sweet and strong smell, this oil is a good source of vitamin A, vitamin B1 and B2 and amino acids. It increases collagen and skin elasticity, which makes it a great choice to combine with vitamin rich essential oils and massage into the skin. It can help keep your skin firm, healthy and young looking.

Borage seed oil is derived from the seed of a starflower plant. The oil is rich in linoleic acid, an essential fatty acid.

This oil is amazing for just about everything, including eczema, dermatitis, breast pain, cancers, diabetes and heart diseases.

Like many carrier oils, this oil is also incredibly hydrating for skin and hair, helping to keep them nourished and healthy.

Castor oil is mainly known for its vitamin E content and is good for healing damaged and dry skin. The texture of this oil is quite unique and unlike most carrier oils, as it is thicker and stickier. This oil has been used all over the world to treat skin related issues, and has even been used to improve the quality of hair and prevent hairfall. For those that want a carrier oil without a very distinct smell, this is a good choice.

Coconut oil not only smells amazing but is rich in Squalenes and vitamin E, which conditions and moisturizes skin and hair and is non comodogenic. Great for both dry and oily skin, and sensitive skin as well. This oil is definitely one of the most celebrated carrier oils out there due to its ability to prevent and improve the appearance of wrinkles, as well as to soothe irritated and flaky skin.

Grapeseed oil is a good source of Omega 6 and Omega 9, making it good for aging skin, It is also an option for acne prone skin due to the fact that it is not overly sticky or pore-clogging, and can help to restore the natural balance of the skin so that it does not produce excess sebum, especially when it is combined with certain essential oils. Depending on what you blend it with, it can benefit almost all skin types, making it a versatile carrier oil.

Jojoba oil is a non fatty oil which contains beneficial ingredients such as vitamin E, vitamin B complex, vitamin C, chromium and zinc. It has a high Iodine percentage as well, which makes jojoba exceptionally useful for healing injured skin or skin with sores, acne, sunburn or rashes. It is great for sensitive skin that is dry, normal or oily.

Macadamia nut oil is a carrier oil derived from the macadamia nut. This oil is a pleasantly rich smelling oil which contains a high amount of vitamin K, vitamin E and omega fatty acids such as omega 6 and omega 3. This oil has been used in skincare and haircare products for many years, and it is proven to benefit the body in numerous ways both by topical application and oral consumption due to its high vitamin and antioxidant content. This oil is better for drier, flaky skin due to its emollient nature.

Olive oil is, perhaps, one of the most well known and celebrated oils in the world. It is used for cooking dishes all over the world, but it is also widely used as a skincare and haircare product. This oil works amazingly as a carrier oil due to its numerous benefits for the skin and body. It is rich in monounsaturated fatty acids and antioxidants.

Peanut oil is another emollient vegetable oil derived from peanuts. This oilis naturally free of trans-fats and cholesterol, and is a source of antioxidants, vitamin E, phytosterols and many more beneficial substances. This oil is known for being great for the health of your skin and hair, but also for your internal organs e.g. your heart.

Pomegranate seed oil is a less well known oil as compared to olive oil, coconut oil, etc. but it is an amazing carrier oil nonetheless. This carrier oil is derived by cold pressing the pomegranate seed, and is naturally high in flavonoids and punicic acid which makes it great for consuming and topical application. It is highly nourishing to the skin due to its high antioxidant content, and it can combat quite a few skin ailments as well as prevent premature aging.

Rosehip oil is derived from the seeds of a specific type of rose. For skincare, this oil has numerous benefits due to its essential fatty acids, vitamin E, vitamin C, B-carotene and more. It is the essential fatty acids that help nourish dry, sun damaged skin and help to fade the marks of burns or scars, as well as reduce wrinkles. Like many other oils, it is also useful for improving the health of your hair.

Sea buckthorn berry oil contains a vast amount of proteins, nutrients, essential fatty acids and vitamins C, A and E that help to make the skin healthier. This oil can be mixed with certain soothing essential oils to treat sunburn or free radical damage, as well as to heal wounds, acne, skin ulcers and the like. It is also a great oil to use on dry, flaky skin prone or eczema sufferers.

Sesame seed oil is derived from the sesame seed and is used in multiple foods, as well as for the skin, hair and body. This oil is a fantastic carrier oil, as it adds many cancer fighting compounds to your essential oil blend, e.g. phytic acid, magnesium, phytosterols, etc. In addition to this, it contains the anti-inflammatory compound called sesamol, which makes it ideal for sensitive or itchy skin. Upon mixing with certaim essential oils, this is a great oil to combat rashes.

Whichever oil you do end up picking will definitely provide you with some great benefits. Carrier oils all have some great moisturizing abilities, no matter what type you pick.

Let's now move on to the next chapter, in which we'll go over the method of blending oils. After that, we'll get the recipes!

Chapter 4 - Blending Essential Oils

In order to receive a variety of benefits, blending essential oils is a great thing to do. However, there are certain rules, precautions and other tips you need to be aware of before you begin, which is why this chapter is an important one.

Let's begin.

Basic rules for blending

One of the most important rules you must be aware of before you try your hand at blending is that you should only blend small amounts of oils when you are starting out. This way, you can figure out what you like and what you don't like without having to waste copious amounts of the expensive oils.

It's a good idea to start by creating a mixture that contains a total of ten drops. So, you could do four drops of one type of oil and four drops of another, and then two drops of a third oil. This is just an example, of course.

Keep the different scents of the oils you are blending in your mind as you do it.

Once you have completed a blend, put a little bit on a cotton ball and sniff it up close, as well as from a distance. If you like it, you can go ahead and create a larger amount.

If you are creating a blend that you desire to use for a certain ailment that you have, then keep in mind the benefits of each oil that you are blending so that you can come up with a blend that has the maximum of the benefit you desire for your issue.

Those are the few basic rules to keep in mind when you're starting out with blending. Next, let's discuss some other tips and precautions.

Blending tips and precautions

As you probably know by now, essential oils can be very irritating and harmful in their undiluted form, which is why it's important to take precautions when blending.

The first precaution that many people seem to overlook is to wear gloves. Yes, I know that gloves can be annoying, but they are a must when it comes to blending.

If even a drop of essential oil that is concentrated falls onto your skin, it will not be pleasant or good for the skin.

Safety glasses are also a good idea, seeing as how essential oils can burn the eyes if they make contact with them.

Another precaution that you might want to take is to perform your blending in a room that is free of children, pets or any distractions. All the open bottles of essential oils would be a recipe for disaster if there was a child or pet in the room.

Another tip to be aware of is that some oils should not be used in blending for aromatherapy at all due to their toxic nature. These oils include parsley herb oil, wintergreen oil, savin oil, wormwood oil, etc.

The final precaution is an obvious one: Do not do your blending in a room that has any sort of fire in it! As I said before, essential oils are flammable.

Those are the main precautions you need to make use of. For the final part of this chapter, I will inform you about the tools that you will need for blending.

Tools required

One of the great things about blending is that you don't need a ton of fancy equipment. However, that being said, there are a few items that you may need to pick up.

The main item you will need is, of course, a bottle-or several bottles, depending on how many blends you wish to make. These bottles need to be small and dark colored with proper caps or lids.

A small glass dropper is also a good thing to have so that you can make it easier to tests the oils and add them together.

You will also need one or two beakers and some stirring spoons.

Safety glasses and gloves are a must, as you will know if you read the previous segment.

You should also have some paper towels on hand to wipe up any spillage.

Finally, keeping some recipe cards to write down your favorite findings is also great so that you can remember how to make your preferred blends again.

That's all you need to know about the basics of blending. Now, we can get on with the fun part-the recipes!

In the following chapters, we'll go over multiple recipes for pretty much every problem you could possibly have.

This is the part of the book that will be of the most use to you.

Chapter 5 - Essential Oils for Illnesses (Recipes)

*Keep in mind that for inhalation via diffusers or steaming, carrier oils are not necessary.

Allergies

Recipe 1:

- 2 tablespoons of jojoba oil (as a carrier)
- 6 drops of eucalyptus oil
- 4 drops helichrysum oil
- 2 drops grapefruit oil

Blend and massage the solution onto irritated area if the allergy is external, or on neck and chest if internal, or inhale by steaming or a diffuser.

Recipe 2

- 2 tablespoons coconut oil
- 6 drops of Roman chamomile oil
- 2 drops peppermint oil
- 2 drops of lavender oil
- 2 drops marjoram oil

Blend, and apply onto the irritated area or inhale.

Appetite balance

Recipe 1

- 2 tablespoons sweet almond oil
- 4 drops grapefruit oil
- 8 drops lemongrass oil

Blend and inhale by whichever technique you like.

Recipe 2

- 2 tablespoons of coconut oil
- 6 drops peppermint oil
- 6 drops lemon oil

Blend and inhale or mix into the bath.

Recipe 3

- 2 tablespoons olive oil
- 4 drops bergamot oil
- 8 drops peppermint oil

Massage onto the neck or inhale via bathwater.

Arthritis

Arthritis is a very common issue among the elderly in particular, but it is one that can be treated with essential oils so that the symptoms are relieved.

Recipe 1

- 2 tablespoons avocado oil
- 6 drops nutmeg oil
- 6 drops juniper oil

Blend and massage into affected area for relief or until the pain starts to subside.

Recipe 2

- 2 tablespoons coconut oil
- 6 drops cypress oil
- 6 drops cinnamon oil

Blend the ingredients and massage into affected area for relief or when the pain starts to subside.

Asthma

Recipe 1

- 2 tablespoons coconut oil
- 6 drops peppermint oil
- 6 drops eucalyptus oil

Blend and mix into the bath or inhale.

Recipe 2

- 2 tablespoons rosehip oil
- 2 drops mandarin oil
- 2 drops rosemary oil
- 8 drops rose oil

Blend and mix into the bath or inhale.

Recipe 3

- 2 tablespoons of sesame oil
- 6 drops of tea tree oil
- 4 drops of lemon oil
- 2 drops of grapefruit oil

Blend and mix into the bath or inhale.

Blood circulation

Recipe 1

- 2 tablespoons of jojoba oil
- 6 drops nutmeg oil
- 4 drops rose oil
- 2 drops marjoram oil

Blend and massage into skin on required areas or add to bath.

Recipe 2

- 2 tablespoons of olive oil
- 4 drops eucalyptus oil
- 8 drops cinnamon oil

Blend and massage into skin on required areas or add to bath.

Recipe 3

- 2 tablespoons of coconut oil
- 6 drops rosemary oil
- 6 drops grapefruit oil

Blend and massage into skin on required areas or add to bath.

These blood circulating recipes can help with a variety of skin issues such as stretch marks and scarring, as well!

Bruises

Many people are prone to bruising easily, and it can be irksome to have to wait weeks for bruises to stop being painful and stop showing so much. Essential oils can help relieve the pain of bruises and make them fade faster.

Recipe 1

- 2 tablespoons macadamia nut oil
- 4 drops juniper oil
- 6 drops peppermint oil

Mix the ingredients properly and massage into affected area with soft hands several times a day and then apply bandage onto the wounds.

Recipe 2

- 2 tablespoons peanut oil
- 4 drops clove oil
- 8 drops eucalyptus oil

Blend and massage into affected area.

Colds

Recipe 1

- 2 tablespoons olive oil
- 6 drops of eucalyptus oil
- 6 drops of lemon oil

Blend and massage into skin (especially near the neck, chest, and abdomen), add to bath or inhale.

Recipe 2

- 2 tablespoons of sweet almond oil
- 4 drops tea tree oil
- 6 drops myrrh oil
- 2 drops peppermint oil

Blend and massage into skin, add to bath or inhale.

Recipe 3

- 2 tablespoons of olive oil
- 6 drops grapefruit oil
- 2 drops cypress oil
- 4 drops chamomile oil

Blend and massage into skin, add to bath or inhale.

Bumps and burns

Burns can occur from contact with heat, steam, hot liquids, chemicals, or the sun. Natural therapies like using essential oil mix can help in wound healing and decreasing pain but for severe burns always need special medical attention.

Recipe 1

- 2 tablespoons coconut oil
- 4 drops mandarin oil
- 8 drops peppermint oil

Blend and massage into affected area or add to bath.

Recipe 2

- 2 tablespoons coconut oil
- 6 drops lavender oil
- 6 drops tea tree oil

Blend and massage into affected area or add to bath.

Recipe 3

- 2 tablespoons sweet almond oil
- 2 drops eucalyptus oil
- 2 drops lavender oil
- 8 drops patchouli oil

Blend and massage into the affected area or add to bath.

Recipe 4

- 20 drops lavender oil
- 4 tablespoons aloe vera oil
- 200 IU vitamin E oil
- 1 tablespoon vinegar

Combine ingredients, and shake well before using, apply as often as possible.

Keep in mind that massaging into the affected area will have a faster and more direct effect on the injury, but adding it to the bath will help with a gradual improvement.

Detoxification

*There is no need for carrier oils in any of these recipes. Dilution with water may be performed if necessary.

Recipe 1

- 4 drops lemon oil
- 4 drops peppermint oil

Blend and inhale via steaming or a diffuser.

Recipe 2

- 4 drops grapefruit oil
- 4 drops tea tree oil

Blend and inhale via steaming or a diffuser.

Recipe 3

- 4 drops carrot seed oil
- 4 drops lavender oil

Blend and inhale via steaming or a diffuser.

If you desire, you may add a carrier oil and add to bathwater, but the results will not be as effective as inhalation without a carrier oil.

Dermatitis

Recipe 1

- 2 tablespoons sesame seed oil
- 4 drops tangerine oil
- 4 drops cedarwood oil
- 4 drops chamomile oil (any variety is fine)

Blend and massage into skin or add to bathwater.

Recipe 2

- 2 tablespoons coconut oil
- 6 drops lavender oil
- 6 drops mandarin oil

Blend and massage into skin or add to bathwater.

Recipe 3

- 2 tablespoons coconut oil
- 2 drops rose oil
- 2 drops vanilla oil
- 8 drops tangerine oil

Blend and massage into skin or add to bathwater.

Notice how most recipes for sensitive issues of the skin use coconut oil—it is the best option for sensitive skin.

Diabetes

It is one of the most common diseases the world is facing today, mostly occurs when the body fails to produce insulin. Genetic and environmental factors play its roll leading to body immune system destroy pancrea's insulin producing cells. The oil recipe below will surely help you to get it in control without using insulin or other invasive methods.

Recipe 1

- Apply 2-3 drops coriander, dill, fennel, equal parts, on the feet in the morning before starting any work, at night apply this oil onto your pancreas.
- 2 drops of coriander, dill, and fennel in capsule, take 1 times a day.

Cypress oil helps treat diabetic neuropathy.

Diarrhea

Diarrhea is better treated if you have purged the bacteria or any parasite causing it. Hydration and essential oils play an important role in treating it.

Recipe 1

- 1 teaspoon thyme oil
- 1 teaspoon tea tree oil
- 1 tea spoon lavender oil
- 1 teaspoon lemon oil
- 1 teaspoon eucalyptus oil

Mix the ingredients mentioned in the recipe and massage clockwise onto your abdomen.

Dry skin

When people's skin does not produce enoigh sebum, the result is dry and flaky skin that feels tight and uncomfortable. To get rid of dry skin, it is a good idea to use a blend of carrier and essential oils.

Recipe 1

- 2 tablespoons borage seed oil
- 10 drops carrot seed oil
- 2 drops mandarin oil

Blend and massage into affected area. Store it in a plastic bottle and use it every time the condition resurfaces.

Recipe 2

- 2 tablespoons coconut oil
- 8 drops lemongrass oil
- 4 drops eucalyptus oil

Blend and massage into affected area.

Ear infection

The ears are a very important part of the body and caution should be used when applying essential oils. The recipe below uses a cotton ball to be inserted into the ear. Use this recipe only if you have got your ear checked.

This is gentle ear relief and cleans the ears without damaging the ear canal.

Recipe 1

- garlic
- mullein
- calendula
- St.John's wort
- tea tree oil
- vitamin E
- olive oil

Shake well and place 3-4 drops in each ear and then insert cotton balls in the ears.

Do not use this recipe if the ear is punctured.

Fever

Recipe 1

- 2 tablespoons jojoba oil
- 6 drops tea tree oil
- 6 drops peppermint oil

Blend and massage into the body (especially the forehead) or add to bathwater.

Recipe 2

- 2 tablespoons rosehip oil
- 6 drops eucalyptus oil
- 2 drops lavender oil
- 4 drops peppermint oil

Blend and massage into the body or add to bathwater.

Recipe 3

- 2 tablespoons rosehip oil
- 6 drops lemon oil
- 6 drops peppermint oil

Blend and massage into the body or add to bathwater.

The reason for including peppermint oil in each recipe is because its cooling sensation makes it the ideal oil for fevers.

Flu

*No carrier oils required unless you wish to add the blend to bathwater. For inhalation, dilution with water is fine.

Recipe 1

- 6 drops lemon oil
- 6 drops tangerine oil

Blend and inhale via steaming or a diffuser.

Recipe 2

- 6 drops peppermint oil
- 2 drops eucalyptus oil
- 4 drops grapefruit oil

Blend and inhale via steaming or a diffuser.

Recipe 3

- 2 drops tea tree oil
- 4 drops ginger root oil
- 6 drops lavender oil

Blend and inhale via steaming or a diffuser.

Gout

Gout is an inflammatory condition, caused by increased amounts of uric acid, which gets accumulated in the areas around joints which contains lubricating fluids. It mostly hurts a lot and occurs commonly in toes and fingers.

This recipe has proved to produce amazing results and can help you get rid of the pain without using any medical treatment.

Recipe 1

- 2 drops of frankincense oil
- 2 drops of basil oil
- 2 drops of geranium
- 2 drops of peppermint oils
- 1 tablespoon of carrier oil

Apply on the affected areas for four hours.

Headache

Recipe 1

- 2 tablespoons sweet almond oil
- 6 drops peppermint oil
- 6 drops chamomile oil

Blend and massage into temples.

Recipe 2

- 2 tablespoons of coconut oil
- 6 drops tea tree essential oil
- 6 drops rosemary oil

Blend and massage into temples

Recipe 3

- 2 tablespoons of olive oil
- 2 drops lemon oil
- 2 drops eucalyptus oil
- 8 drops clove oil

Blend and massage into temples.

Inhalation is also an option for these recipes if massaging does not do the job.

Immune system booster

Recipe 1

- 2 tablespoons of grapeseed oil
- 6 drops lemon oil
- 6 drops grapefruit oil

Blend and add to bathwater for a citrus filled boost. Inhalation is also an option.

Recipe 2

- 2 tablespoons jojoba oil
- 2 drops lavender oil
- 4 drops peppermint oil
- 6 drops lemongrass oil

Blend and add to bathwater or inhale via a diffuser or spray.

Recipe 3

- 2 tablespoons jojoba oil
- 8 drops tea tree oil
- 4 drops tangerine oil

Blend and add to bathwater or inhale via a diffuser or a spray.

Indigestion

Recipe 1

- 2 tablespoons sweet almond oil
- 4 drops lemon oil
- 2 drops grapefruit oil
- 6 drops peppermint oil

Blend and massage into abdomen or chest area, or inhale via bathwater or a diffuser.

Recipe 2

- 2 tablespoons sweet almond oil
- 4 drops ginger oil
- 2 drops lemon oil
- 6 drops chamomile oil

Blend and massage into abdomen or chest or inhale via bathwater or a diffuser.

Recipe 3

- 2 drops rose oil
- 8 drops eucalyptus oil
- 2 drops grapefruit oil

Blend and inhale via a diffuser.

Itchy skin

Itchy skin, whether it is from a rash or some other skin issue, is highly bothersome. To soothe the itchiness, try out some of these great recipes.

Recipe 1

- 2 tablespoons coconut oil
- 6 drops tea tree oil
- 4 drops peppermint oil
- 2 drops carrot oil

Blend and apply using a cotton swab, apply 2-3 drops of this mixture to affected area. Apply as often as possible.

Recipe 2

- 2 tablespoons olive oil
- 6 drops eucalyptus oil
- 6 drops helichrysum oil

Blend and apply using a cotton swab, apply 2-3 drops of this mixture to affected area. Apply as often as possible.

Recipe 3

- 2 tablespoons rosehip oil
- 6 drops nutmeg oil
- 6 drops oregano oil

Blend and apply to affected area. Apply as often as possible.

Knee pain

Knee pain can be caused by many things and basically means the inflammation of joints. Symptoms include pain ,swelling, redness, tenderness,and rigidity of joints. It stops you from doing any physical activity which makes the problem even worse.

There are many essential oil blends which can help you relieve the pain.

Recipe 1

- 20 drops of sweet marjoram
- 15 drops of cinnamon leaf
- 15 drops of lavender oil
- 10 drops of peppermint oils
- 2 tablespoons of fractionated coconut oil

Mix all the ingredients in a plastic bottle and apply it onto any painful area, if applied on large patches on the body then mix it further by 2 tablespoons of carrier oil.

Liver cleanse

When it comes to liver cleanses, citrus oils are the way to go, which is why I've included at least one citrus oil in each recipe.

Recipe 1

- 6 drops lemon oil
- 6 drops grapefruit oil

Blend and inhale via a diffuser or steaming.

Recipe 2

- 2 drops lemon oil
- 2 drops peppermint oil
- 8 drops bergamot oil

Blend and inhale via a diffuser or steaming.

Recipe 3

- 2 drops rose oil
- 2 drops tea tree oil
- 2 drops chamomile oil
- 6 drops lemon oil

Blend and inhale via a diffuser or steaming.

Migraine

Migraines should be treated similarly to headaches, but with more potent blends.

Recipe 1

- 2 tablespoons coconut oil
- 6 drops peppermint oil
- 6 drops tea tree oil

Blend and massage into temples or inhale via steaming.

Recipe 2

- 2 tablespoons olive oil
- 6 drops eucalyptus oil
- 6 drops clove oil

Blend and massage into temples or inhale via steaming.

The reason I am suggesting steaming over a diffuser is so that you get a stronger kick from the oils to help relieve the migraines.

Muscle pain

Recipe 1

- 2 tablespoons coconut oil
- 6 drops nutmeg oil
- 6 drops rosemary oil

Blend and massage into affected area or mix into the bathwater.

Recipe 2

- 2 tablespoons of grapeseed oil
- 2 drops peppermint oil
- 2 drops marjoram oil
- 8 drops chamomile oil

Blend and massage into affected area or mix into the bathwater.

Recipe 3

- 2 tablespoons grapeseed oil
- 6 drops sandalwood oil
- 4 drops clove oil
- 2 drops cinnamon oil

Blend and massage into affected area or mix into the bathwater.

All of these oils are known to relieve sore, achy muscles.

Psoriases

It is a painful skin condition which causes swelling in large areas of the skin and results from skin cells producing too quickly. The skin gets covered in white scales.

People with psoriases have benefited by using essential oil blends as yet there is no proper treatment for it. It can be caused by emotional stress, poor diet ,hormonal changes, vitamin D deficiency, genetics, poor liver function.

You can use the following essential oil recipe to help you relieve the pain.

Recipe 1

- 20 drops of chamomile oil
- 20 drops of apricot kernel oil
- 20 drops of jojoba oil
- 20 drops of avocado oil
- 5 tablespoons of carrier oils

It can also help you get rid of dandruff, acne and in treating wounds, burns, boils.

Respiratory Function

During cold and flu season this recipe is recommended.

Recipe 1

- 2 drops lemon oil
- 2 drops lime oil
- 2 drops peppermint oil
- 2 drops rosemary oil
- 2 drops eucalyptus oil

Blend all the essential oils together and apply it onto the chest, back and on the inner thighs to improve circulation.

Rosacea

Rosacea is yet another skin disease, which gets very irritating and affects many people. It is difficult to cure. Symptoms are redness and swelling around the cheeks and face intermittently, may also spread to neck, chest, ears, nose, and scalp, annoyance, irritable behavior with blood vessels visible on the face.

Using these few essential oils can improve your condition and help you heal from this disease quickly.

Recipe 1

- 1 teaspoon castor oil as it reduces swelling
- 1 drop german chamomile
- 1 drop helichrysum

Mix the ingredients and store it in a plastic bottle, apply using a cotton dab on the affected areas gently. Try not to rub as it can aggravate the redness and swelling.

Snoring

Snoring can be triggered by many different underlying problems such as the anatomy of the mouth and sinuses, alcohol consumption, allergies , cold and body weight.

Combine the recipe below in the smallest amount to see if it helps you out. It is sure going to make a change.

Ingredients:

- 25 drops geranium
- 25 drops lavender
- 25 drops marjoram
- 10 drops cedarwood
- 8 drops eucalyptus radiate
- 8 drops sweet basil
- 2 tablespoons pure water

Use peppermint oil if it happens due to nasal congestion, due to this oil's anti-inflammatory properties.

Stomach ache

Recipe 1

- 2 tablespoons olive oil
- 6 drops lemongrass oil
- 4 drops ginger oil
- 2 drops peppermint oil

Blend and massage into the skin near the abdomen or add to bath.

Recipe 2

- 2 tablespoons olive oil
- 6 drops vanilla oil
- 6 drops eucalyptus oil

Blend and massage into the skin near the abdomen or add to bath.

Recipe 3

- 2 tablespoons olive oil
- 3 drops patchouli oil
- 4 drops lemon oil
- 5 drops bergamot oil

Blend and massage into the skin near the abdomen or add to bath.

Inhalation can also be performed with these blends.

Sunburn

Keep in mind that citrus oils should be avoided when one is sunburnt!

Recipe 1

- 2 tablespoons coconut oil
- 2 drops eucalyptus oil
- 6 drops peppermint oil
- 4 drops tea tree oil

Blend and massage into affected area.

Recipe 2

- 2 tablespoons coconut oil
- 6 drops lavender oil
- 6 drops chamomile oil

Blend and massage into affected area.

Recipe 3

- 2 tablespoons coconut oil
- 2 drops rose oil
- 10 drops tea tree oil

Blend and massage into affected area.

Adding aloe Vera gel to your essential oil mixtures is also a great way to soothe sunburns.

Sweating

Many people have issues with excessive, uncontrollable sweating. Essential oils can help with that.

Recipe 1

- 2 tablespoons coconut oil
- 6 drops lemongrass oil
- 6 drops lemon oil

Blend and apply to areas where excessive sweating occurs.

Recipe 2

- 2 tablespoons coconut oil
- 6 drops tea tree oil
- 4 drops peppermint oil
- 2 drops clary sage oil

Blend and apply to areas where excessive sweating occurs.

The citrus oils will eliminate the odor of sweat while the other oils will help reduce the sweating in general.

Tendonitis

Tendonitis is a form of painful, inflammation condition of the tendons. It is caused by doing excessive exercise or sitting in the same position for many hours, injuries or built up inflammation. It can cause a lot of pain. It is more common in people with 40 plus age. It mostly involves surgical treatment but using this essential oil blend can help you relieve the immense pain accompanied by tendonitis.

Recipe 1

- 25 ml of olive oil
- 5 ml of Neem oil
- 30 drops of lavender oil
- 20 drops of marjoram
- 10 clary sage
- 5 german chamomile
- 3 drops of peppermint oils

Mix this well and apply to hands and toes daily until the pain lessens.

Let's now move on to the cosmetic uses of essential oils, and what recipes can be used in that aspect.

Chapter 6 - Cosmetic Uses of Essential Oils (Recipes)

Acne

Recipe 1

- 2 tablespoons coconut oil
- 2 drop pine oil
- 4 drops tea tree oil
- 2 drops sweet orange oil
- 4 drops eucalyptus oil

Blend and massage onto affected area.

Recipe 2

- 2 tablespoons coconut oil
- 2 drops grapefruit oil
- 4 drops yarrow oil
- 6 drops ginger oil

Blend and massage onto affected area.

Recipe 3

- 2 tablespoons coconut oil
- 4 drops valerian oil
- 2 drops tangerine oil
- 2 drops rose oil
- 4 drops lemon oil

Blend and massage onto affected area

Recipe 4

- 2 tablespoons coconut oil
- 6 drops tea tree oil
- 6 drops lemongrass oil

Blend and massage onto affected area.

Baby care

While there's no prove that essential oils can improve your baby's health, there are studies showing that lavender oil can relax and calm baby. The recipe given below soothes the baby and treats eczema and skin irritation and will help you take better care of the baby.

Recipe 1

- 1 cup of organic olive or apricot or kernel oil (softer fragrance and good for sensitive skin)
- 2 tablespoons calendula flowers
- 2 tablespoons chamomile flowers

There are two ways to make this recipe.

Fast way: According to the recipe above, infuse over heat in a double boiler, then add calendula and flowers with the heat continuously going on from low to medium for at least an hour or until the oil has started to turn yellow.

Slow way: Put the calendula and chamomile in a glass jar and pour oil over it, keep it tightly lidded placing it in a cool, dark place and shake daily for 6-8 weeks.

Cellulite

Cellulite is the fat deposits under the skin. This recipe is a citrus massage oil, smells great and helps to improve skin circulation.

Recipe 1

- 0.25 cup hazelnut oil
- 0.25 cup jojoba oil
- 10 drops cypress essential oil
- 8 drops grapefruit essential oil
- 7 drops cedarwood essential oil
- 5 drops orange essential oil
- 5 drops lime essential oil
- 5 drops lemon essential oil

Mix all the ingredients and shake thoroughly before using.

Chapped lips

Chapped lips are a bothersome issue that almost everyone faces in the colder seasons. Fortunately, essential oils and carrier oils are amazing for replenishing moisture back into the lips!

Recipe 1

- 2 tablespoons of pomegranate seed oil
- 6 drops of rose oil
- 6 drops vanilla oil

Blend and apply using the index finger. Store in a container.

Recipe 2

- 2 tablespoons castor oil
- 6 drops mandarin oil
- 6 drops carrot seed oil

Blend and apply using index finger. Store in a container.

Deodorant

As you learned in the previous chapter, citrus oils are great for deodorizing, but so are a few other oils.

Recipe 1

- 2 tablespoons rosehip oil
- 6 drops lemon oil
- 4 drops sandalwood oil
- 2 drops rosemary oil

Blend and apply to underarms.

Recipe 2

- 2 tablespoons jojoba oil
- 2 drops clary sage oil
- 2 drops jasmine oil
- 2 drops Ylang-ylang oil
- 6 drops peppermint oil

Blend and apply to underarms.

Recipe 3

- 2 tablespoons coconut oil
- 6 drops sweet orange oil
- 6 drops cinnamon oil

Blend and apply to underarms.

All of these mixtures can be applied to any part of the body that requires deodorizing.

Facial cleanser

Finding a cleanser that removes dirt from your skin without being harsh and drying is a difficult task, which is why it is a good idea to create your own cleanser with the help of essential oils.

Recipe 1

- 2 tablespoons pomegranate seed oil
- 6 drops pine oil
- 6 drops tea tree oil

Blend and store in a bottle or jar. Take a dime sized amount and apply softly onto the face with hands.

Recipe 2

- 2 tableapoons peanut oil
- 6 drops mandarin oil
- 2 drops juniper oil
- 4 drops eucalyptus oil

Blend and store in a bottle or jar. Take a dime sized amount and apply softly.

Foot care

Feet are a part of the body that we often neglect, but which we should give some extra care. Instead of using artificial and chemical laden moisturizers, why not try a natural blend of oils to care for your feet?

Recipe 1

- 2 tablespoons castor oil
- 4 drops carrot seed oil
- 8 drops mandarin oil

Blend and apply to soles of feet, massage gently.

Recipe 2

- 2 tablespoons coconut oil
- 6 drops lemon oil
- 6 drops peppermint oil

Blend and apply to soles of the feet, massage gently.

Hair

Recipe 1

- 2 tablespoons coconut oil
- 6 drops lavender oil
- 6 drops Ylang-ylang oil

Blend and smooth onto hair and massage into scalp.

Recipe 2

- 2 tablespoons olive oil
- 6 drops rosemary oil
- 2 drops tangerine oil
- 2 drops cedarwood oil
- 2 drops lemon oil

Blend and smooth onto hair and massage into scalp.

Recipe 3

- 2 tablespoons coconut oil
- 6 drops sweet orange oil
- 6 drops lemongrass oil

Blend and apply to underarms.

These oil mixtures may be kept on the hair for a few hours or overnight before being washed off. The best part about these recipes is that it is not only the essential oils, but the carrier oils that are also nourishing the hair!

Hair loss

To increase hair growth and stop the balding process, this recipe is sure going to help you by increasing circulation and stimulating the scalp.

Recipe 1

- 4 tablespoons of apple cider vinegar
- 20 drops of carrot essential oil
- 10 drops of rosemary essential oil
- 1 tablespoon for ice cold water

Massage onto your scalp before going to bed and rinse it in the morning.

Nails and skin

The composition of nails and skin and hair is similar, so the recipes can be interchanged if you'd like.

Recipe 1

- 2 tablespoons sweet almond oil
- 6 drops lemon oil
- 6 drops tea tree oil

Blend and massage into nails or skin.

Recipe 2

- 2 tablespoons argan oil
- 6 drops peppermint oil
- 6 drops rose oil

Blend and massage into nails or skin.

Recipe 3

- 2 tablespoons jojoba oil
- 2 drops grapefruit oil
- 6 drops eucalyptus oil
- 4 drops lavender oil

Blend and massage into nails or skin.

Rashes

Rashes can be very irritating and prove to be irritating if not treated properly. This recipe would be good to apply to the rash directly or by applying it onto a piece of cloth or paper tape and then dabbing it onto the rash.

Recipe 1

- 5 drops chamomile or 10 drops lavender
- 2 drops peppermint oil
- 3 tablespoons baking soda
- 2 cups water (or use peppermint tea instead)

This recipe can be made in a tea form or applied topically.

Varicose veins

Varicose veins are nasty, swollen veins located on the leg as a result of poor circulation and decreased elasticity in the walls of the veins.

Recipe 1

- Two large bowls
- 3 drops lavender
- 3 drops geranium

Add 3 drops of lavender oil in cold water, place both feet in cold water in five minutes, next add 3 drops of geranium to hot water and place feet in hot water for five minutes.

Warts

Warts are describes as being small skin lesions, circular in shape, viral in nature. Epidermal layer of skin is affected by the warts, this virus is contagious and can be passed by contact, by sharing personal items such as razors, towels, e.t.c. Warts can be extremely painful and mostly treated by surgery but given below is a very authentic recipe for treating warts at home.

Recipe 1

- 20 drops oregano
- 20 drops frankincense
- 20 drops tea tree
- 20 drops medieval mix
- Raw organic apple cider vinegar

Add essential oils to a bottle and fill it with apple cider vinegar.

Using a cotton swab, apply 2-3 drops of this mixture on the warts.

Chapter 7 - Essential Oils for Improving Welfare (Recipes)

Anxiety Relief and Calming

Recipe 1

- 2 tablespoons jojoba oil
- 6 drops tea tree oil
- 2 drops peppermint oil
- 4 drops chamomile oil

Blend and add to bathwater or inhale without carrier oil via steaming. May also be massaged into the skin.

Recipe 2

- 2 tablespoons jojoba oil
- 4 drops cedarwood oil
- 4 drops jasmine oil
- 4 drops rose oil

Blend and add to bathwater, steam or massage into skin.

Recipe 3

- 2 tablespoons olive oil
- 6 drops marjoram oil
- 6 drops sandalwood oil

Blend and add to bathwater, steam or massage into skin.

Recipe 4

- 2 tablespoons olive oil
- 2 drops cinnamon oil
- 2 drops lemon oil
- 8 drops peppermint oil

Blend and add to bathwater, steam or massage into skin.

Recipe 5

- 2 tablespoons coconut oil
- 2 drops lemongrass essential oil
- 10 drops Ylang-Ylang essential oil

Blend and add to bathwater, steam or massage into skin.

Recipe 6

- 2 tablespoons coconut oil
- 2 drops jasmine oil
- 2 drops lemon oil
- 8 drops tangerine essential oil

Blend and add to bathwater, steam or massage into skin.

Steaming will give you an instant boost, but the slow relaxation of baths is also pretty great.

Depression

Recipe 1

- 2 tablespoons coconut oil
- 6 drops bergamot oil
- 6 drops Jasmine oil

Blend and massage into skin or add to bathwater.

Recipe 2

- 2 tablespoons rosehip oil
- 6 drops chamomile oil
- 6 drops marjoram oil

Blend and massage into skin or add to bathwater.

Recipe 3

- 2 tablespoons rosehip oil
- 6 drops cedarwood oil
- 6 drops vanilla oil

Blend and massage into skin or add to bathwater.

Recipe 4

- 2 tablespoons olive oil
- 2 drops lemon oil
- 2 drops bergamot oil
- 8 drops yarrow oil

Blend and massage into skin or add to bathwater.

Energy level

To boost the overall energy level in your environment, use the following oil blend.

Recipe 1

- 8 drops grapefruit
- 4 drops lavender
- 4 drops lemon
- 2 drops basil essential oil

Blend and massage into skin or add to bathwater.

Fatigue

Recipe 1

- 2 tablespoons jojoba oil
- 6 drops clove oil
- 2 drops grapefruit oil
- 4 drops eucalyptus oil

Blend and massage all over body or add to bathwater.

Recipe 2

- 2 tablespoons coconut oil
- 6 drops cinnamon oil
- 6 drops rosemary oil

Blend and massage all over body or add to bathwater.

Recipe 3

- 2 tablespoons coconut oil
- 4 drops peppermint oil
- 4 drops geranium oil
- 4 drops bergamot oil

Blend and massage all over the body or add to bathwater.

Healthy Immune Response

This works really in spring and summer and helps strengthen your immune response.

Recipe 1

- 2 drops lavender oil
- 2 drops lemon oil
- 2 drops peppermint oil

Mix the ingredients well and apply on the pulse points, neck and feet.

Insomnia

For insomnia, a drop or two of the essential oils mentioned below can be put on pillows or bed sheets (without a carrier oil) as well.

Recipe 1

- 2 tablespoons sweet almond oil
- 6 drops chamomile oil
- 4 drops eucalyptus oil
- 2 drops yarrow oil

Blend and massage into body.

Recipe 2

- 2 tablespoons coconut oil
- 2 drops vanilla oil
- 2 drops valerian oil
- 8 drops lavender oil

Blend and massage into body.

Recipe 3

- 2 tablespoons grapeseed oil
- 6 drops sandalwood oil
- 6 drops Ylang-ylang oil

Blend and massage into body.

Nausea

Nausea can be stimulated by various health conditions such as constipation, anxiety, parasites, indigestion, foodpoisoning, stomach flue, pregnancy, or motion sickness. There are different oils for different stimulants. This recipe given below is especially designed for nausea caused by indigestion.

Recipe 1

- 4 drops ginger
- 4drops lavender
- 3 drops peppermint
- 5 teaspoon carrier oil (argan, coconut, sesame, sweet almond, jojoba ,grapeseed, macademia)

Combine carrier oil with essential oils in a small bowl, gently massage over the abdomen in a clockwise direction.

Oral care

Recipe 1

- 2 tablespoons coconut oil
- 6 drops clove oil
- 6 drops peppermint oil

Blend and apply to teeth, gums or any affected area in oral region.

Recipe 2

- 2 tablespoons coconut oil
- 6 drops lemongrass oil
- 6 drops peppermint oil

Blend and apply to affected area.

Stress

Recipe 1

- 2 tablespoons olive oil
- 6 drops chamomile oil
- 6 drops cedarwood oil

Blend and apply to body, bath or inhale.

Recipe 2

- 2 tablespoons rosehip oil
- 2 drops bergamot oil
- 8 drops chamomile oil
- 2 drops peppermint oil

Blend and apply to body, bathwater or inhale the mixture.

Recipe 3

- 2 tablespoons rosehip oil
- 6 drops rose oil
- 6 drops lavender oil

Blend and apply to body, bathwater or inhale the mixture.

Recipe 4

- 4 drops roman chamomile
- 3 drops lavender
- 2 drops clary sage
- 2 drops geranium
- 1 drop Ylang-Ylang

Blend and apply to body, bathwater or inhale the mixture.

Uplifting

Sometimes, whether it's due to hormone fluctuations or some events in our lives, we tend to feel down. Fortunately, the use of certain oils has been proven to help create an uplifting and energizing feeling!

Recipe 1

- 6 drops pine oil
- 6 drops lemongrass oil

Blend and inhale via steaming to freshen up and feel energized.

Recipe 2

- 2 tablespoons rosehip oil
- 6 drops nutmeg oil
- 6 drops chamomile oil

Blend and massage into the neck and chest area.

Workout

To have a more energetic workout, use the following oil mix to increase vigor and performance.

Recipe 1

- 2 drops of peppermint
- 2 drops of grapefruit essential oil

Take about 120ml of water and these ingredients in a spray bottle and shake it well. Spray it on all exposed areas of the body just before you are about to begin your workout.

Let's move on to the next chapter.

Chapter 8 - Essential Oils for Weight Loss and Anti-Aging (Recipes)

Weight Loss

Citrus is a major fat burner, making it great for weight loss, as well as several other essential oils.

Carrier oils will not be needed in these recipes.

Recipe 1

- 2 drops grapefruit oil
- 2 drops lemon oil
- 8 drops ginger oil

Blend and inhale via steaming or a diffuser.

Recipe 2

- 6 drops peppermint oil
- 4 drops bergamot oil
- 2 drops cinnamon oil

Blend and inhale via steaming or a diffuser.

Recipe 3

- 2 drops chamomile oil
- 2 drops sweet orange oil
- 2 drops sandalwood oil
- 6 drops lemongrass oil

Blend and inhale via steaming or a diffuser.

Anti-aging

These recipes are more skincare related, for mature individuals in particular.

Recipe 1

- 2 tablespoons coconut oil
- 2 drops lemon oil
- 10 drops tea tree oil

Blend and massage into skin.

Recipe 2

- 2 tablespoons argan oil
- 6 drops grapefruit oil
- 2 drops rose oil

Blend and massage into skin.

Recipe 3

- 2 tablespoons grapeseed oil
- 6 drops sandalwood oil
- 6 drops tea tree oil

Blend and massage into skin.

Chapter 9 - Essential Oils for Home and Pets (Recipes)

Air fresheners

Recipe 1

- 6 drops lemon oil
- 6 drops peppermint oil

Blend and place in diffuser.

Recipe 2

- 2 drops lemon oil
- 2 drops grapefruit oil
- 8 drops chamomile oil

Blend and place in diffuser.

Recipe 3

- 6 drops lavender oil
- 6 drops rose oil

Blend and place in diffuser.

Recipe 4

- 4 drops eucalyptus oil
- 8 drops bergamot oil

Blend and place in diffuser.

Candles

When it comes to candles, start out by creating a smaller candle to test it out before creating a full sized one.

Recipe 1

- 6 drops lemon oil
- 6 drops peppermint oil

With this ratio, the candle will smell refreshing and clean.

Recipe 2

- 6 drops chamomile oil
- 6 drops lavender oil

This is an example of what a calming and soothing candle could be like.

Feel free to use the same ratios when creating a full sized candle.

Cleaning supplies

Peppermint, eucalyptus and tea tree are some examples of purifying essential oils. Here are some recipes to create cleaning products from essential oils!

Recipe 1

This can be used to clean combs and brushes.

- 10 drops tea tree oil
- 10 drops eucalyptus oil

Blend and soak brushes for 20 minutes before rinsing and drying.

Recipe 2

This can be used to remove dried up gum.

- 10 drops orange oil
- 10 drops lemon oil

Blend and apply to area with a cotton ball.

Recipe 3

This can be used to clean windows.

- 4 tablespoons of water
- 5 drops lavender oil
- 5 drops lemongrass oil

Blend and use to wipe down windows.

Floor cleaner

Recipe 1

- 10 drops lemon oil
- 10 drops tea tree oil

Blend and use to wipe down floors.

Recipe 2

- 10 drops lavender oil
- 10 drops grapefruit oil

Blend and use to wipe down floors.

Mosquito repellant

Recipe 1

- Two tablespoons coconut oil
- 5 drops citronella oil
- 7 drops tea tree oil

Blend and apply to entire body.

Recipe 2

- Two tablespoons coconut oil
- 6 drops tea tree oil
- 6 drops peppermint oil

Blend and apply to entire body.

Recipe 3

- Two tablespoons coconut oil
- 8 drops eucalyptus oil
- 4 drops lavender oil

Blend and apply to entire body.

Recipe 4

- Two tablespoons coconut oil
- 2 drops clove oil
- 2 drops lemongrass oil
- 8 drops spearmint oil

Blend and apply to entire body.

Pet's products

Recipe 1

This recipe is great to remove pet odor.

- 6 drops lemongrass oil
- 6 drops orange oil

Blend and diffuse into air or spray onto area where scent lingers.

If you wish to apply directly to pet, make sure to dilute heavily with a carrier oil.

Recipe 2

This recipe is one that can boost the health of your dog or cat by treating infections. Again, this must be heavily diluted and mixed with a carrier oil if applied directly.

- 6 drops bergamot oil
- 2 drops eucalyptus oil
- 4 drops chamomile oil

Recipe 3

This recipe is great for pain relief for cats or dogs from arthritis, sprains, etc.

- 6 drops ginger oil
- 6 drops peppermint oil

All of the oils in this segment are safe for the use of cats and dogs as long as they are properly diluted.

Conclusion

With that, we have reached the end of the book. I hope it was an enjoyable read, and I wish you the best of luck on your journey to a healthier, calmer, younger looking and better–feeling version of yourself.

Essential oils are truly one of the most beneficial substances available which are not only natural and free of harmful chemicals but are often more effective than the commercial products that you find at most stores.

Keep in mind that you always need to be on your guard when using essential oils, as they may occasionally cause allergic reactions in some people.

Sensitive individuals or pregnant women should consult a doctor if they plan to use essential oils on a regular basis, just to ensure that it is okay.

By reading this book, you have obtained all of the necessary information to improve the quality of your life.

Use the knowledge in this book to your advantage, and don't let it go to waste!

Now, no more hesitating. Just get up and get started!

Thank you for reading!